HYPNOBIRTHING

Welcome your Little Angel in Pure Peacefulness

(Second Edition)

♣

Dr. Melissa Keane

Introduction

I want to thank you and congratulate you for downloading the book, *"Hypnobirthing"*

This book has actionable information about Hypnobirthing.

Despite being the most natural thing in the world, the fear of childbirth is something lingering at the back of every woman's mind. Unfortunately, society in general, and other women who have gone through childbirth in particular, only exacerbate the problem by telling their stories of horror to expectant first time mothers.

Childbirth is painful; that much is true. However, it is also beautiful and natural. Since it is natural, even without the fussiness of modern medicine that once Labor commences offers unnecessary props such as multiple cervical checks several times a day (or even an hour), the denial of food to the woman, and painful, often inflammatory IV drips that cause numbness in the arm, the body of a woman is perfectly capable of birthing.

Do not construe this to mean modern medicine be dammed! No! Hurrah for modern medicine: it has helped thousands of women give birth in a safe environment that ensures proper care and maximum safety for the mother and child. However, for millennia, women have been giving birth unaided by modern, borderline intrusive medical procedure such as elective C-sections to a point where the female brain and body have developed such unison that each knows what it has to do to facilitate childbirth.

While every woman is different and has her opinion on how childbirth should be, if you are one of the women who believe childbirth should be as natural as God or the universe intended it, if you believe the myth of 'unbearable childbirth pain' should lay on its death bed, Hypnobirthing is something you should try.

What is Hypnobirthing? This book will elucidate Hypnobirthing and teach you about the great difference Hypnobirthing could make in your next childbirth irrespective of whether you decide to have your child at home, through midwifery, or at the hospital under the careful watch of a doctor.

Thanks again for downloading this book. I hope you enjoy it!

Dr. Melissa Keane

The information herein is offered for informational purposes solely, and is universal as so. The presentation of the information is without contract or any type of guarantee assurance.

The trademarks that are used are without any consent, and the publication of the trademark is without permission or backing by the trademark owner. All trademarks and brands within this book are for clarifying purposes only and are the owned by the owners themselves, not affiliated with this document.

Table of Contents

Motherhood

A woman becomes a mother when she first learns that she has conceived. The bond you start sharing with the tiny zygote is so intense and powerful, that from that moment onwards, you can feel it in your heart. The nine months of pregnancy (or less sometimes) is the phase when you see yourself growing, not just around the belly, but also as an individual. You start feeling the movements and the hiccups too.

The beauty of motherhood is the journey you go through from conception to birth and to raising the child. Each one's experience varies a lot. The experience you have with one child may not be the same with another.

"It takes a village to raise a child." This phase is rightly used when it comes to parenting. The challenges we face during this phase can be many and a little bit of encouragement from your partner and family or from fellow mothers and parents is usually very helpful. Despite the challenges we face, there is no equal joy a mother can experience than that of seeing a wonderful creature she can fearlessly bring out in this world.

Conception & Pregnancy

Conception and pregnancy is the first step to motherhood. The joy of conception is unexplainable in terms of how a woman feels. Each one has a different experience and each pregnancy is different. Quite often, women go through a complicated pregnancy. The journey at this point can be very painful and a lot of precaution needs to be taken when the pregnancy is difficult. It is best to listen and take guidance from your obstetrician to help you through this process.

Challenges in Conception

Many couples face a real struggle with conception. They may have some medical problems because of which they cannot conceive and that can create a very negative mindset. The world is changing. Science has managed to come up with various solutions with regards to conception and how you can get pregnant. There are numerous choices out there that you can choose from to make it happen. It is important to determine the real problem or medical condition (for both men and women) and come up with the best possible solution. Fertility centres and fertility hospitals will be the best resource to provide you with the solutions required for you.

Before we get to a point of discussing how to use Hypnobirthing, we will start by understanding what it is first.

Hypnobirthing 101: Understanding Hypnobirthing

Most women have heard such traumatic stories of painful childbirth that when they get pregnant, the mind and body develop such a negative imagery and belief of the whole prospect that when it's time to give birth, the body is a wound up ball of stress and immense tension.

Can you guess what happens next?

Well, because the mind has adopted and accepted the "childbirth is hell week multiplied by infinity" mentality—even first time mothers who have never gone through childbirth— the body tenses up and the pain they expected manifests multiplied manifolds. Despite the fact that the body knows what to do, how to do it, and when, the disconnect between the brain and the body is so profound that in some instances, administered pain relief medication fails to ease the pain.

What if I told you that childbirth does not have to be as excruciatingly painful as the horror stories make it out to be? What if I told you that, through a simple antenatal program called *Hypnobirthing,* you can, like Anna Wall of Austin Texas, be so relaxed through childbirth that even though you shall experience everything, hear everything, and see everything, you can drift off into peaceful slumber mid-contraction? Would that arouse your interest? Would a natural, almost painless, yet ecstatic childbirth interest you? If it would, you should try Hypnobirthing.

What is Hypnobirthing?

Although just now beginning to gain popularity in America and the United Kingdom, Hypnobirthing is not what you would call a new concept. In fact, the concept dates back to the 1940s when Grantly Dick-Read, Obstetrician extraordinaire, published a book, _Childbirth without Fear_, in which he introduces the idea of hypnotherapy for childbirth, a notion that uses hypnosis to reduce and even eliminate childbirth pain altogether.

It is through Grantly's work that the current propagator of natural childbirth, Marie Mongan, came to learn about using hypnosis to reduce pain and remain calm during childbirth. So what is Hypnobirthing? Well:

"Hypnobirthing is the use of hypnosis and relaxation techniques as aids in the childbirth process to make the process as painless (remember that the nature of pain depends on perception) as possible."

Hypnobirthing functions on the premise that since childbirth related pains are often a result of a negative mindset towards the prospect—thanks to societal norms—fear and tension, by engaging in hypnotherapy, something that involves breathing techniques, relaxation of the muscles, body, and mind, and hypnosis, it is possible to reduce, or even eliminate Labor pains.

It is important to understand that Hypnobirthing doesn't guarantee a pain free birth, but it does guarantee that it will be more comfortable and gentle and you will be more in control of your body while giving birth. That being said, there are thousands of women who have had a pain free birth due to the hypno-birth practice, but everybody is different and has different levels of pain threshold.

So how did the concept of Hypnobirthing begin? That's what we will discuss next:

A Brief History of Hypnobirthing

Today, because of the popularity and effectiveness of Hypnobirthing, women across the United Kingdom are flocking Hypnobirthing classes by the droves not compelled or attracted by some flashy ad on telly, but through word of mouth. This shows just how effective this childbirth approach is.

How Hypnobirthing came to be so popular is thanks to Marie Mongan, a follower of Grantly's work, and through her childbirth experience, led to what has now become *Hypnobirthing™–The Mongan Method.* Marie's story is an amazing one that shows how the determination of one woman and her desire to have a natural childbirth can cast such an influence on modern day society.

Married at a time when creating a childbirth plan or having a husband in the delivery room was unheard, when Marie went into Labor with her first child, she told the attendant her intent to have a natural childbirth. The attendant, thinking she was coocoo, smirkingly insisted that soon enough, and like the thousands of women who gave birth at the hospital, she would be screaming in agony, begging for pain relief medication.

The nurse left her alone in a room (at the time, husband were societally disallowed from being in the delivery room) that had a clock she could use to time her contractions. Marie, a proponent of Hypnobirthing as described in Grantly's work, practiced the hypnosis and breathing techniques she had practiced all through her pregnancy and before long, her body signaled the need to push. She rang the nurse and as would be expected, after the nurse rancorously examined, she saw the baby's head crowning.

In panicked haste, the nurse bundled her onto a trolley and rushed her to the delivery room where Marie went through the rigmarole of modern day childbirth: a hard surgical couch, legs in stirrup, and an IV drip with God knows what kinds of drugs. In Marie's case, instead of an IV, they strapped her wrists to the couch and even though she had communicated her desire to have a natural childbirth, they chloroformed her and the next thing she knew was coming to only to find a baby, her baby, lying in a cradle besides her. She felt furious, disappointed, and upset. Unfortunately, the same thing happened with her second child.

When Marie was pregnant with her third child, she did not want to go through what she went through with her first two children. Although she wanted to have her baby at home, she could not and instead, explicitly directed her obstetrician to give orders that the attendants allow her to give birth in the natural way she has been preparing for throughout her pregnancy.

When she finally went into Labor, she was a spectacle because she was doing something new, and unlike the first two times, her daughter came into the world through a calm, drug free, yet painless natural delivery that left many thunderstruck.

Many years later when her daughter and two of her friends, now all grown up, conceived, she developed Hypnobirthing™– The Mongan Method, which she used to help them experience, painless, natural, and calm births. The success of these three births was the tidal wave the method needed to become a phenomena and soon after, hypnotherapists, Medical people, and Childbirth educators from all over the place, including Canada and Australia, were thronging Marie's office to learn about her method.

Marie late founded the Hypnobirthing™ institute in America as her method continued to spread through word of mouth in America and Canada. She later went to England where she taught her method where like in America and Canada, the method spread through word of mouth and today, thousands of women across the United Kingdom are advocates of the method, justifiably so because the method works and women want to give birth the natural way.

If pregnant and would like to try Hypnobirthing for a natural, painless birth, you may be a bit skeptical, not because you are unsure of your body's ability to know what to do, but because modern medical norms, society, and the numerous birthing horror stories you have heard/read, have led you to believe that unaided, painless childbirth is a myth.

In the next section, we shall allay your skepticism by discussing how Hypnobirthing works, look at case studies, and then outline a simple Hypnobirthing hypnosis technique you can practice all through your pregnancy to get yourself—body and mind—ready for a natural, painless birth.

Labor

All through your pregnancy, you will probably go through mixed emotions of excitement, happiness, fear and anxiety. All these feelings of fear and anxiety are natural but it doesn't have to be that way. You don't need to be in a negative frame of mind just anticipating what it might be like when you go into labor. There are many ways by which you can combat that feeling and have a wonderfully smooth pregnancy. As already mentioned above, Hypnobirthing is a great option. A lot of women have practiced Hypnobirthing for multiple pregnancies and some have their first labor to compare it to, and most of them have stated that their experience with Hypnobirthing and the labor has been much smoother than expected. They were able to have a calm and relaxed mind, without any negative feelings and go through their labor smoothly. Some required medical intervention and had to undergo a C-section, but even those women claim to have had a very calm and peaceful delivery, while being able to control their anxiety and have their body in control. Even if you are not practicing Hypnobirthing, labor can be handled well. Having a positive mind frame and also having the right support system besides you can make things easier.

Challenges during labor

Preterm Labor – Having labor contractions before 37 weeks is considered to be preterm labor. Preterm labor can be risky for the mother and the baby, especially the baby as its lungs may not be fully developed or the body is unable to generate enough heat to keep the baby warm. The baby and the mother can undergo distress and it can prove to be very dangerous for the both of them. At this point, it is important to stay calm and focused. You have to be positive and understand that many preterm babies survive with little medical intervention and that it is possible to have a healthy baby. If you have the backup of Hypnobirthing during this phase, can you imagine how helpful it may prove to be to you? A mother who is already expected to be worried and probably anxious and scared, will actually be able to stay calm and focus on her baby. The breathing techniques will send positive energies to the baby and make sure that the body is not is stress and the placenta is getting enough oxygen throughout.

Prolonged Labor – Unfortunately for some, labor can go on for days. It is called "failure to progress." During this phase, both the mother and the baby are at a risk of some danger and the baby may go into distress. The heartbeat may drop and medical intervention may become inevitable. Mostly, in such cases, it is seen that due to the prolonged labor and the mother not being able to cope with the pain, babies can become distressed. The stress hormones in the mother's body naturally increase and she isn't able to control the outcome. In such times, Hypnobirthing can be very helpful. We have talked to many mothers who have had prolonged labor and they swear by Hypnobirthing. They claim to have had much more control over their bodies and go through days of labor and still manage to have a natural birth, although some have said that they needed to undergo a C-section eventually, but even then, they were able to stay calm throughout the process.

Abnormal Presentation – Abnormal presentation refers to the part of the baby that will appear fist through the birth canal. A few weeks before the due date, the fetus drops lower into the uterus and ideally for labor, the baby has to be positioned head-down. The baby's head leads the way through the cervix into the birth canal. Some babies, however, do not change position and present themselves with the buttocks first. This is known as the breech position. Breech position is normally seen before the due date and many babies usually turn into the head-down position eventually on their own. In a case where that doesn't happen, it is still possible to have a normal birth. With the help of Hypnobirthing, you can definitely birth vaginally because of the various benefits it provides.

How to be prepared, when the water breaks & the pains kick in?

There is no need to panic when the water breaks; usually you have enough time to reach the hospital on time to deliver the baby. If you are having a home birth or water birth, it is essential to stay calm. The key is to stay as relaxed as possible. Probably, your birth partner will be in a state of panic, but you have to stay focused.

What do you do when the baby finally arrives?

The joy of motherhood really begins after the baby is here. The first time you see your baby, how you feel when you hold the baby is a feeling that you may have never experienced before. However, there are times when mothers don't feel any different and may need some time to accept the birth of their child and that is okay too. Don't be too hard on yourself, wondering why you don't feel elated like most mothers do. It applies to the father as well. It is alright to cut yourself some slack and ease into the zone of parenting.

Once the baby is out, you can choose to tell your midwife to either give the baby immediately to you, or clean the baby first. It is ideal to have the baby on your chest immediately, as this skin to skin will help you bond with the baby and stimulate your milk supply. The father can also provide skin to skin to the baby in case the mother is unable to for any reason. It is of utmost importance to breastfeed the baby immediately or within an hour of being born. You can try the breast crawl as well, or just latch the baby on to your breast. Do not worry about your milk supply, as the first milk, i.e. colostrum, is enough to satiate the baby's hunger until your milk starts. Babies cry for many reasons. Don't always assume that the baby is hungry and feel discouraged that your milk supply is low. Continue feeding the baby on demand and this in turn will help you increase your supply. The equation is simple, more demand equals more supply. Keep yourself well hydrated and continue eating a well balanced diet.

You need to keep some things in mind before getting the baby home. You will have to prepare for everything before the baby arrives. This includes things like having the car seat ready to take the baby home. You also need diapers and clothes. In the case that you have a pet, make sure that he/she is prepared before introducing the baby to the pet. Pets can get overwhelmed with this new member in the family and that is why it is important to prepare the pet a few days in advance. Once the baby is born, and you are still at the hospital, take the baby's used clothes or blanket home for the pets and let them sniff them from a distance. This way they are familiar with the baby by the smell when they arrive home.

Raising a baby

Raising a baby can be very overwhelming. The constant crying and waking can get you and your partner overly tired and exhausted. Try to find your own fun in these times if possible. There will be times when you may just want to escape from the situation, but knowing that 'This Too Shall Pass' will help you both go a long way. It is important to know that the baby needs you more than ever. Its tiny body is also going through changes and this big new world may be scary. Keep the baby close and you will not regret it. Listen to your instincts and believe in yourself.

Hypnobirthing can be very useful even after birth. You have already learnt all the breathing techniques and you have your calming relaxing music with you. While you are breastfeeding or putting the baby down for a nap, listen to this music. It will keep you calm and help your baby stay calm too. In the same way as Hypnobirthing will help you go through the pregnancy and birthing, it can also help you with raising your child.

Short Break to Leave a Review?

If you are enjoying this book so far, may I ask you to leave a review on Amazon? It will take you one minute and it will help me a lot to improve the quality of this book. It just has to be an honest review!

And you know what? Amazon usually gives you a heads up every time an author performs major changes and updates in the interior of a book!

Having said that, I would really appreciate you help!

Post Partum Depression

Many mothers suffer from Post Partum Depression. There are certain symptoms that you may experience while going through depression and it is very important to analyse yourself as early as possible and sort it out. It is a feeling where you feel completely overwhelmed and suppressed and you feel like "Motherhood is not meant for me, I can never do it." The feeling of guilt, anger may be present and the fact that you put so much pressure on yourself can cause PPD and, if not recognized in time, can unfortunately put you through circumstances that can be dangerous to both you and the baby. It is, however, very treatable. There are ways you can get it sorted out by just talking to your doctor or Obgyn and get a prescription to help you through it.

However, if you have practiced Hypnobirthing, this can be fought more easily. It is false that the mother who has gone through a Hypnobirthing class never faces PPD, but it is definitely helpful in terms of keeping you calm and your nerves in place. That is why Hypnobirthing is gaining more and more popularity across the world as most parents, especially mothers, have to go through this all alone without any support system and need to be calm and handle everything single handedly.

At the end of the day, motherhood is a blessing. It is the most fulfilling feeling in the world. You ought to feel proud of how well you have managed to go through pregnancy and birthing, and believe that you are doing your best to raise your baby well. A mother is God's gift to us. She puts herself second to all her baby's wishes and thrives on doing her best for the baby. Be proud of yourself and keep moving ahead with a positive attitude.

How Hypnobirthing Works, Its Benefits & Effective Hypnobirthing Techniques

It is easy to understand why many women are, at first, skeptical about Hypnobirthing and how it works, if it works at all. This section of this Hypnobirthing guide is going to describe how Hypnobirthing works and why it works, discuss some of the benefits of Hypnobirthing, and then to top this section, we shall engage in a thorough discussion of the various ways through which you can practice Hypnobirthing. You are in for a treat:

How Hypnobirthing Works

As we stated earlier, although now a public phenomenon—thanks to celebrity advocates such as Jessica Alba and Tiffani Thiessen—self-hypnosis for birth, what we now know as Hypnobirthing, is not new. In fact, experts in this field are quick to point out that self-hypnosis for childbirth has been in existence for centuries, long before Grantly's research.

With that said however, only in the last three decades has the prospect gained acclaim and wide use to a point where, throughout the world, but majorly in the U.S., UK, Canada, and Australia, women are considering hypnosis for childbirth and integral part of the antenatal process. Today, hypnosis for childbirth is so popular that other than Hypnobirthing™–The Mongan Method, there are other Hypnobirthing programs such as The Leclaire Hypnobirthing Method, Hypbirth, and Hypnobabies.

Even though most of these programs vary in their offerings, most have the same concept: *use hypnosis, breathing, and relaxation techniques to help women intending to have a natural childbirth overcome the fear that incites physical pain in childbirth.*

Our bodies have a system called the fight-or-flight system/mechanism. When we are fearful, this system releases into the body stress hormones called catecholamines; the work of these hormones is to slow the rate of digestion and speed up the heart thereby increasing blood flow to the arms of legs (the things you need to fight or flee).

When we are fearful, more so of the childbirth pain we 'believe is forthcoming,' the fight-or-flight system, because it is automatic, depletes blood flow to the uterus, which as you may guess, hinders the Labor process, which then leads to uterine pain.

Hypnotherapy works by ensuring full body and mind relaxation, something impossible when the fight-or-flight system is active. When you hypnotize yourself into replacing the fear of childbirth with relaxation, instead of releasing stress hormones into the blood stream, the body releases relaxation and feel-good hormones such as oxytocin, endorphins, dopamine, and serotonin, and prostaglandins—Labor hormones. Together, these hormones lead to immense relaxation of all bodily muscles and a state of calm and comfort.

The last few decades have been very stressful for women in terms of childbirth. The fear and the agony of just thinking about childbirth is more difficult than the actual childbirth, which make this natural process seem traumatic.

In ancient times, we humans were much more relaxed and calm during childbirth, as the process was considered to be extremely normal. Women from the community would gather around the mother and create a calm environment for her to birth in. The role of the father was also more crucial and involved at the time. He would build a birthing room for the wife and let her relax on the bed. Once labor pain began, he would sit leaning behind her and help her by pushing the abdomen so that the baby would come out smoothly. Naturally, having the husband beside her and supporting her was a great relief for the wife. He would then hold the baby once it was born and cut the umbilical cord and give the baby to the mother.

When it comes to what Hypnobirthing teaches, you will have to take a Hypnobirthing course/class irrespective of which Hypnobirthing method you are following. Most of these classes, in particular, the Hypnobirthing™–The Mongan Method, consist of five classes of 2½ hours each. The cost of the course depends on your location and the service provider; normal costs are $275 (£ 213) to $350 (£ 271).

The course shall teach you various breathing and visualization techniques that all aim to help you visualize and envision an easy painless birth where your cervix willingly opens wide to facilitate effortless childbirth. In some instances, thanks in part to the advent of technology, some hypnotherapists are willing to offer online courses, CDs, and even Skype consults.

Once you learn the hypnosis, relaxation, visualization, and affirmation techniques, you and your partner should practice them each day of your pregnancy. For instance, when Wall, the woman we mentioned earlier, went through the course, she learnt and practiced affirmations such as "I am relaxed and so is my baby," "my baby is just the right size and my body can comfortably and painlessly accommodate and deliver her." This helped her delver he baby in an easy, painless way.

When you practice such affirmations, your subconscious mind will accept them, and then use them to replace the fear of birth, which will reduce, or even eliminate the pain you experience when it is finally time to bring your child into this world.

Another thing some, not all, of these classes shall teach you is how to replace specific words our minds associate with pain. For instance, when Anna was going through the class and daily practice, her hypnotherapist taught her how to reject common word references associated with painful or difficult childbirth and in their place, use words that have a lesser negative connotation. Instead of saying contraction or pain, she learnt how to use words such as 'surge' and 'sensation' in their place.

Most Hypnobirthing techniques, whether Hypnobirthing™–The Mongan Method, or Hypnobabies, teach the same thing with very limited variations. A good example of this is hypnobabies that although teaches hypnosis for childbirth, teaches mothers to be how to self-hypnotize with their eyes open all through the process and in some instances, provides antenatal training that moves beyond self-hypnosis.

Role of your Obstetrician in Hypnobirthing

If you have a birth plan, it is important that you discuss it with your Obstetrician. You have to clear all your plans with the Obstetrician in advance so that there is no confusion when the time comes. Whether you intend to have a natural birth, a C-section or whether you choose to take an epidural and also if you have been practicing Hypnobirthing, all these things need to be conveyed to your doctor and your midwife well in advance. If you have been practicing Hypnobirthing, you will be much calmer and more in control of your body, hence it is important that this is conveyed to them in advance and explained, so that they know what to expect and take your calm and relaxed stature seriously and know that you have it all under control. Involving your birth partner in this plan is also very important, as they can be the ones to insist on your plans if at all you are not in a position to do so.

Now that we have a firmer understanding of what Hypnobirthing is, how it works, and why it works, let us look at some of the benefits of using Hypnobirthing:

The Benefits of Hypnobirthing for the Baby, Mother, and Father

Research has shown that any stress a pregnant mother experiences affects the baby's development. In this respect, Hypnobirthing, which as we have seen, revolves around relaxation and measured breathing, can be very beneficial.

As a point of note, in the weeks before birth, a baby's brain is rapidly developing. Any stress or anxiety on the mother's part, as various research studies have shown, is bound to have a long-term effect on the baby's brain development. By disrupting stress and anxiety, which is what deep breathing, relaxation, and hypnosis does, you ensure nothing compromises your baby's development before and after birth.

It is very difficult for the mother and father to stay relaxed during childbirth. For many years now, the stress and tension of birthing has increased to such an extent that it only brings panic and utter fear in the minds of the mother as well as the family. To be honest, even the doctor's don't really prepare you. They do not tell you techniques on how to be calm during labor and explain how important it is to be so. If a woman is feeling immense stress while giving birth, the body releases a hormone known as adrenaline. This adrenaline rush signals the brain that there is something wrong and potentially harmful to the mother and the baby and signals that their life could be in danger. This stress and body reaction can lead to the mother progressing towards stress labor, which in turn can stress the baby's heartbeat and compel the doctor to take immediate action such as a C-section.

The response to this adrenaline is that it tends to divert the blood away from the uterus and send it to the other parts of the body, which clearly do not need this rush of blood. This is known as the flight or fight response. This is a great mechanism of the body and the brain to react to an alarm that the body is producing but it is absolutely not good for a quick and comfortable labor as the natural process of birthing gets hindered by this process. The oxygen that the uterus and the cervix needs to have for a calm and comfortable birthing experience is pushed to other parts of the body, which do not need this oxygen at that point.

For the Mum and Baby

Hypnobirthing, as the title of this sub section suggests, has benefits not only for the baby, but for the mother and the father as well. Let us discuss these benefits:

Deep Relaxation: Hypnobirthing promotes deep relaxation, which at its very core, is the foundation for a positive and happy pregnancy. Hypnobirthing main goal is to teach you how to enter into an instance state of deep relaxation. When you are relaxed, the body creates a natural sense of wellbeing.

Through guided imagery and relaxation techniques practiced throughout pregnancy, when the time to deliver your baby, because you know how to relax instantly, Kerry Tuschhoff from hypnobabies says that through deep relaxation, you can "anesthetize" your body. This means less pain and angst as you deliver your baby.

When relaxed and in a natural anesthetized state, the effects will trickle down to the baby you are bringing into the world because as research has shown, during Labor, babies can feel everything the mother feels. When you are relaxed, meaning feel good and anesthetic hormones are flowing through your veins, this effect will trickle down to the baby and your baby is bound to come into this world calm. When you and the baby are calm all through Labor, your husband is also likely to be calm because in most instances, Hypnobirthing involves both couples practicing affirmations and manifestation together, and when Labor comes, the husband guides the wife through repeating the affirmations and manifesting a calm birth.

Rewires your Subconscious Mind: The subconscious mind is very powerful (a super computer); so powerful that through its power, we form associations with words and specific events. For instance, when most women think of Labor or childbirth, because of their perception towards it, a perception formed and housed in the subconscious mind, they think of unbearable pain and anguish.

When you start practicing Hypnobirthing strategies such as hypnotism and affirmations, because when you are in a hypnotic state, your subconscious mind is malleable, and as such, through affirmations, you can rewire it into thinking differently about the various words associated with Labor and childbirth.

For instance, most women attach negative inferences to the word "contractions." Through Hypnobirthing, you learn to replace this word (and its meaning to you) with another positive and less negative word such as "birthing waves." This rewires your subconscious mind and because when in a hypnotized state, it is pliable, instead of associating contractions with pain, you start associating them with waves that come and go.

If you start practicing this strategy early in your pregnancy, you can get to a point where through imagery and visualization, you can associate this wave with pleasure (like surfing a wave), which as you can guess—and because natural, painless childbirth is a mind's game—would lead to an easy, painless, almost ecstatic childbirth.

Trust: Hypnobirthing, at its very core, is all about getting you to trust your body's natural ability to know what to do when and in which manner to bring into this world your baby without much angst. It does so by helping you dispel the fear of birth. When you are no longer fearful of birthing waves, you begin trusting your body and when you trust your body, you know you are capable of giving birth in a painless way.

Further, by practicing positive affirmations and visualizations, you shore up your self-belief. For instance, when you practice an affirmation such as "I trust my body to know how to birth my child in a painless way," your subconscious mind adopts this affirmation as the truth. Because of this, when the time to deliver comes, because we attract that which we profess and focus on, your body will know what to do to bring your child into this world.

Although we may have discussed this only in passing, Hypnobirthing is also very beneficial to babies not just in the weeks before birth, but after birth too.

For one, because the mother will be relaxed, stress and anxiety free all through pregnancy and Labor, the baby's development will be optimal because as research has shown, stress during pregnancy does affect child development.

Secondly, most babies delivered through conventional births where the mother believes birthing is painful instead of a natural psychological and physiological process experience trauma. Hypnobirthing helps reduce this trauma because when the mother is stress and anxiety free all through the pregnancy, and calm instead of tensed during childbirth, the baby will come into this world in a calm and gentle manner.

Babies whose mother practice Hypnobirthing techniques also have a higher Agpar scores thanks to the calmness of their birth. An Agpar score is a measure of how well the baby is doing immediately after birth and then five minutes later.

For the Dad/Birth Partner

For the dad or the birth partner, the advantages of Hypnobirthing revolve around cementing the familial bond and making the partner feel part of the process. Because most Hypnobirthing classes are partner based, learning how to stay calm, confident, and in control throughout the birth process is a plus for all involved.

Now that we have looked at the benefits of Hypnobirthing, let us look at some ways through which you can practice Hypnobirthing.

Effective Hypnobirthing Techniques

NOTE: While this book shall outline the best way to hypnotize yourself for birth, practice deep breathing and visualization for a pain free and pleasurable birth, if you can afford it, attend a Hypnobirthing class where you can learn firsthand. The five classes (this is standard for most Hypnobirthing programs) are 2½ hour long each but their effects will stay with you long after birth.

With that in mind, let us now discuss various Hypnobirthing strategies and techniques:

How to Self-Hypnotize for Birth

The Self-hypnosis for birth technique we shall discuss here is very similar to guided meditation for birth. As such, and to make this practice your go to when Labor waves start, practice this technique every day of your pregnancy. This practice involves elements of hypnosis, meditation, and elements of guided imagery (visualization) guaranteed to help you relax and accept the possibility of a comfortable and painless birth.

It is wise to point out that—and this goes back to the need to attend Hypnobirthing classes if you can afford them—practicing self-hypnosis works best when firstly, an experienced hypnotherapist guides you through the process to a point where you form associations with certain cues and can do it all on your own. If you cannot afford the Hypnobirthing classes, you can use this YouTube video

Once you can get into a deep state of relaxation on cue, here is how to self-hypnotize:

Step 1

Start by getting comfortable. For this purpose, you can either sit or lie down in a pregnancy-friendly position at a place that affords you quiet for 20-30 minutes. While the idea here is to remain lucid all through the process, if you drift off to sleep, that is also ok; if you practice this strategy for a substantial amount of time before your due date, you will have figured out how to self-hypnotize without falling asleep.

Step 2

Set a goal for the session. Here, you need to choose what you want to focus on in a particular self-hypnosis session. This will make the session that much more focused and thus effective. You can choose any of the following:

- Restful sleep

- Freedom from fear and anxieties

- A painless/comfortable birth

- A healthy baby

- Shorter Labor, etcetera

Attaching a goal to your hypnosis session gives your subconscious mind a goal.

Step 3

Choose a focal point. This can be a point in the room. It can also be internal with your eyes closed. With your eyes closed (or looking at your focal point), breathe deeply (Diaphragmatic breathing). Take a deep breath in through the nose to a count of 4 and out to a count of 8. The in and out breathe should be loud enough (at first) that someone in close vicinity can hear.

Continue breathing in this manner and with each inhale, repeat a positive affirmation as you concentrate on positive energy and pure intentions.

As you exhale, visualize yourself letting go off all stress, fear, and tension accumulated anywhere on your body. Continue breathing in this manner and in your mind, repeat affirmations such as "I'm deeply relaxed," "I'm letting go of all tension," or "I'm positive."

If you had chosen to keep your eyes open, they will start feeling heavy; you can let them close naturally.

Step 4

Once deeply relaxed and your body feels tension free, visualize your body being as light as a feather and getting lighter with each in and out breath. This step is open to personalization. Depending on your goal for the session, you can choose to visualize your body filling with positive warmth and light as you inhale. Visualize the light permeating every bit of your being: the head, the shoulders, the arms, the core and your baby, thighs, calves, hands and toes: everywhere.

Step 5

Now visualize yourself at the top of a staircase that has 10 stairs. The staircase is leading to a meadow: an oasis of peace. Compel yourself to descend the stairs and with each step you take, visualize each stair number in your mind and yourself drifting further into a sea of deep relaxation.

At the fifth stair, stop for a moment to enjoy the deliciously enticing and laxative smells coming from the meadow below. Tell yourself you are entering a meadow where everything is just as you want it, where your baby is safe, where you are capable of birthing in a painless way.

As you descend the last 5 steps, immerse yourself in the gloriousness of the meadow and everything it brings with it; feel completely at ease, relaxed, and at peace and one with yourself, the universe, and your baby: visualize going through the birth you want to experience: peaceful, calm, and pain free.

Step 6

Once in the meadow, visualize your goal for the session as a big treasure box. For instance, if your goal for the session is "overcome the fear of painful childbirth," imagine yourself going to that box and as you open it, repeat a positive affirmation such as "my Labor shall be relaxed and comfortable" and as you do this, see yourself experiencing a painless childbirth. Notice and feel the peace and elation you feel as you bring your child into this world in an effortless and painless manner. Repeat your affirmation several times.

Step 7

Joyously make your way back to the stairs (prance around and feel like a princess) and begin ascending each stair one a time and as you do, carry with you all the feelings and sensations you experienced while in the meadow.

Step 8

When you get to the 10th step, open your eyes and become fully conscious only fully refreshed, relaxed, and positive.

This hypnosis technique is very powerful and if you practice it as detailed here all through your pregnancy (preferably once or twice daily), you will carry everything you experience in the meadow to your chosen birthing location and experience the birth you envision.

Hypnobirthing Breathing Techniques

The breathing techniques taught in Hypnobirthing classes are some of the most effective and important tools you could have at your disposal as a mother preparing for birth. The key to using these breathing techniques is to make sure you are completely relaxed, which you can do using the hypnosis technique above.

NOTE: As you practice these breathing techniques, always remember to rest your tongue on the upper part of your mouth behind your upper teeth. This ensures you release all the tension in your jaw region and thus, tension in your pelvis.

The breathing techniques that are used during Hypnobirthing are very crucial and are recognised as the most important tool to stay calm and composed during labor. Here are some of the relaxation techniques you can practice.

Relaxation Breath

It is very important that you relax yourself completely before you begin with the relaxation breathing exercise. Your face and body need to be very relaxed and calm. Rest your tongue behind your front upper teeth. This ensures that you are not holding any tension between your jaws. Tension in the jaw can lead to tension in the pelvis. Place one hand on your heart and one hand on your belly. While breathing, close your eyes and imagine that you are filling a large balloon. Take a deep breath, inhaling through your nose very gently for as long as you can and then exhale gently through your nose. You can also visualize yourself being lifted up in the air when you breathe in, and gently descending and reconnecting with the Earth when you breathe out. Remember, during labor, you will experience contractions and surges that can take your breath out of balance.

This technique will help you stay focused during labor and get you re-centered for your next surge and sail smoothly through the contractions.

Breathing through the Surge (contraction)

Remember that Hypnobirthing is all about changing your perception towards birth and the perceived pain (which is why we replace a word such as 'contraction' with 'surge').

As you inhale through your nose (remember, you are engaging in diaphragmatic breathing), visualize filling an inner balloon with air and take as deep a breath as you can and inflate the balloon as much as you can).

As you breathe out, direct the energy of the breath down, and as you visualize the balloon deflating, also visualize any tension in your pelvis as a wave that lifts you up gently, reaching a peak, and then gently coming down. Imagine yourself riding this ecstatic ride.

It is this breath that will provide you the most support during labor. Practice this breath, from early on in your pregnancy and during the birth process because, it puts you into a good habit of connecting with your baby and breathing in a relaxed way during labor. The surge breath involves a really long slow inhale of breath, breathing up through your nostrils using your diaphragm (belly breathing) for a long count and as long as you can inhale. You can use a counting technique while practicing this breath. Some people find that very helpful. But you don't need to be attached to how many numbers you can count up to. It may differ every day depending on how you feel (What you need to focus on is your breath and slow inhalation), and then slowly releasing the breath outwards through your nose, by focusing on your baby. It is really important that you don't hold your breath. You can use that breath many times during your surge. For example, if you're having a one minute surge you can take probably three surge breaths, which means that you are inhaling to the count of 10 counts during one of the three surge breaths and exhaling to the count of 10 counts.

Surge breaths are one of the most important and valuable breaths. It is increasingly valuable as your labor progresses and your surges increase in strength and intensity, where you take as many surge breaths as you need. What is really valuable when you're taking your surge breath is to add in a special visualization. Some mothers like to imagine or visualize that they are filling a balloon. As they take a deep breath in, they imagine the balloon being filled up with air (you can give a colour to the balloon) and the air slowly releasing as you take a deep breath out, while the balloon slowly deflates as the energy is directed down towards the baby. As stated above, some mothers like to imagine that they are floating in the air while they breathe in and slowly re-connecting with the ground and the baby as they breathe out, slowly and uniformly. You can imagine some warm, beautiful and relaxing waves and colors. You can imagine yourself floating like a cloud and fill it with colors of your choice. You can also imagine the waves of the ocean, because the rhythmic flow of the ocean is so beautifully in contact with the surge breathing as the waves also reach a peak and then slowly fall down as they get into contact with the ground towards the shore.

Breathing through Bearing Down

As you did in the previous breathing exercise, breathe through the nose but this time, make the in breathe quicker and the outer one as long as you can while directing the breath down and out. As you breathe out, the out breath should resonate at the back of your nose and the muscles in your stomach should feel as if you are giving them a light workout.

Now that we have looked at the various reasons why you should take Hypnobirthing classes and discussed the various ways you can hypnotize yourself and breathe through the surges and bear downs, let us look at general Hypnobirthing tips that upon practicing, shall help you have an easy, positive pregnancy.

Birth Breath

Birth breath is not something that you can practice a lot before birthing. It is important that you have an understanding that once you become fully dilated the baby still has a way to never get down the birth path to be born. So the birth breath really involves trusting your body and following the lead of your body with a shorter inhale of breath and a longer exhale of breath down into your body. It is normally demonstrated as breathing in strongly, and breathing out through your mouth, while you involve your voice to get the breath out of your body and the energy to pass on to your baby.

J Breathing

J breathing is one of the many Hypnobirthing tools you can use to help you feel really calm and in control when you birth your baby. The reason this technique of breathing is called J breathing is because you're breathing your baby downwards into your body. This breath is very specific so it's good for a specific phase of labor, so you will have gone through your labor and birth in such a way that your cervix opens beautifully and, after a point, your baby will come down and put some pressure on your pelvic floor and you will feel an involuntary urge that you want to push. You may feel a pressure to poo as well. This is a good sign, it means that you may actually not want to poo but the baby is putting enough pressure on your rectum and has gently travelled down to the birth canal. The J breath is the most appropriate tool to help you stay calm. Unlike the other breathing techniques, J breathing helps you really push the baby down.

How to practice J breathing:

Relax your shoulders and your jaw line. Breathe in through your nostrils and into your throat. It is a technique where you're opening up your throat so that you can feel the air travel down. Place a hand on your throat very gently, to bring your attention there and gently breathe out through your throat. In this method of breathing, you can hear your breath through your throat, as it is a very noisy breath. You don't have to count the breath. Breathe in slowly and the exhale is also as long and as slow as you can make it. In this breath, you have to imagine that you are breathing all the way down to your baby and then past your baby down to your vagina. Consciously keep all the muscles on your face relaxed and breathe right down to your vagina. You may feel a bit of tension in your throat as you are engaging that muscle for this technique of breathing in a different way. You may also experience a little bit of heat and tension in your belly during this process, which is normal. You may also choose to chant OM while breathing out during J breathing. Chanting OM has no religious backing to it. However, if you are not comfortable, you may skip this step. You may need your partner, mother or sister or anyone who is there to support you to help remind you to practice J breathing during this phase of labor, in case you forget about it and the other techniques are not working for you.

Tips on How to create self-hypnosis
Breathing Method 1

Breathe in to 4 counts; breathe out to 4 counts. Repeat this as many times as required, but a minimum of 15 times a day.

Note - It is required to be seated in an upright position to perform these breathing exercises, but these simple breathe in and breathe out exercises can be done anywhere, whether you are standing or sitting. Keep a calm relaxed face and begin.

Breathing Method 2

Saying positive things to yourself while breathing can help build a clear frame of mind. Slowly and steadily, you will be going from a stressed state of mind to a calmer and in control state of mind. Saying things like "I am calm," "I am confident," "I can do it" really make a big difference as to how you see your journey from there on. By controlling the breath, you automatically lower your stress adrenaline levels and the panic hormone that could interfere with your smooth birthing process. The happy hormone that is the Oxytocin is immediately released when you are positive and feeling good and confident about yourself.

A Unique Special Place

Allow your mind to find yourself a unique and special place where you are relaxed, feel calm and comfortable. It could be any place in the world. Say, for example, as a child you liked to go and sit under the big tree in your back yard while you listened to the bird's chirp and the squirrels run. Choose that place, and, in your imagination, sit there and feel. Work with your imagination. Imagine different colors and scenarios. You subconscious mind cannot tell the difference between real and imagination. This lets you disassociate yourself with any feeling of negativity or stress related to your birthing experience. You will eventually love to visit that place and even during labor, this can be practiced for smooth sailing.

Listening to a Hypnobirthing Audio

If possible get yourself a Hypnobirthing CD even if you can't attend the class. There are many audios available online that you can choose to listen to. When you are visualizing, you are daydreaming. You can also let your husband or life partner listen to this audio as they are, whether you believe it or not, in a very difficult state of mind as well. They are scared and tensed just like you and this process will help your partner to a great extent.

The Best Tips for a Happy and Positive Pregnancy

A happy pregnancy is one where instead of being fearful of the birthing surges, you eagerly anticipate the day, hour, and minute you get to deliver and hold your baby in your arms for the first time. It is one where rather than envision pain, you visualize a calm and painless birth full of elation. The last section of the last chapter has taught you how to use Hypnobirthing techniques such a hypnosis, visualization, and affirmations to achieve that.

In this section of the guide, we are going discuss tips that shall help make your pregnancy and happy one. Remember to couple these tips with the strategies discussed above.

1: Enroll In Hypnobirthing and antenatal Classes

While this book has outlined the various ways you can practice Hypnobirthing at home, it is also important to note that the knowledge and hands-on experience you will receive from attending a class where you will learn from an experienced hypnotherapist alongside other mothers shall prove invaluable.

Enroll in a class as early as possible (take your partner along) and once you learn the various strategies, practice them every day.

Enroll in a class as early as possible because most of these classes fill up fast while some course such as the Bradley method can run for up to 12 weeks.

It is also wise to enroll in an antenatal class where you can ask all the Labor related questions you may deem pressing. As you take these classes, do not be afraid to ask seemingly stupid questions: your peace of mind is more important than appearing stupid. Question your midwife or doctor on things such as a natural birth, epidurals and cesarean sections, the different stages of Labor, best nutrition for pregnancy, and other such relevant questions. The idea here is to be as informed as possible.

2: Don't Be a Couch Potato

While this is conventional knowledge, it is still super important. Motion is one of the most important ways to eliminate tension within the body. If you relegate yourself to the couch, just because you are carrying a baby in you, you will be dooming yourself and your baby and lovingly welcoming a difficult, painful pregnancy.

Exercise is a good way to stay active. However, do not become an exercise buff who is overly obsessed with maintaining a specific weight. Engage in moderately taxing exercise such as yoga, easy jogging (in the first and early second trimester), and walking. Remain consistently active throughout the pregnancy and above all, remember to listen to your body: if an exercise feels wrong, stop.

3: Watch What You Eat and Use

This is fundamentally important: what you eat will determine your health as well as the health and wellbeing of your baby. Consume a balanced diet consisting of more fruits, veggies, proteins and complex carbs, and minimal, if any, amounts of simple carbs such as diet sodas, white rice, artificial sweeteners, and the likes.

Reduce your exposure to environmental (cleaning products and such) as well as food and drinks toxins. In all, eat real foods and if you can, use natural products for all your cleaning and personal care purposes.

4: Adopt the Right Mindset

This is at the core of Hypnobirthing. You have to let go off all your perceived notions of how pregnancy and Labor should be and instead, reinforce, through hypnosis, visualizations, and affirmations, how you want your pregnancy and Labor to be. Of importance to remember is that our bodies are intelligent enough to know that pregnancy is natural and thus, the body shall do everything necessary to accommodate the pregnancy without causing you much pain because the body hates pain and will do everything necessary to overcome it, including releasing natural anesthesia.

5: Prioritize

As a mother to be, whether this is your first pregnancy or you have been through several, you have a home to manage and a lot to tick off your To-do list before your baby comes into this world. If you fail to prioritize everything you have to do, you will feel overwhelmed, which will welcome stress into your life.

Create a list of all the things you need to do and then prioritize these in order of importance. If something is not important, strike it off your list or if it has any bearing on your pregnancy, delegate it to your partner or members of your extended family if you have one.

6: Savor Every Bit of It and Create Enjoyable Memories

Most pregnant women often forget that pregnancy ought to be enjoyably memorable. Most are so concerned with the impending pain of Labor that all they wish is for the nine months to whiz by as fast as possible. Avoid this as much as you can.

Instead, take deliberate action and dedicate time and money to enjoying your pregnancy. Go for picnics, movie dates, fun adventures in nature, and engage in anything else that brings you happiness and is memorable. Document—through pictures and videos—as much of the pregnancy as you can because before long, 9 months will have passed and you will miss the feeling of being pregnant.

7: Meditate

This is very important. Meditation is the ultimate way to internal satisfaction and happiness with yourself and your life. Further, scores of research studies prove that meditation eases tension, stress and anxiety. Here, you can choose to focus on your breath, phrase (mantra), or music. Choose a way to meditate (there are thousands of ways to meditate) and then practice it every day for serenity and happiness.

8: Pamper Yourself

Who doesn't feel happy after a pampering session? Whenever the opportunity presents itself (you can deliberately create the opportunity), pamper yourself. Reward yourself for being such a strong women who is doing everything in her power to give birth to her baby in a calm and peaceful manner. Take yourself out on a spa date; eat your favorite dessert as you lazy around the couch for a few hours watching your favorite chick flick movie, etc.

9: Visualize

The mind cannot differentiate between the real and imagined; to it, they are all the same. This makes visualizations very powerful. When you visualize yourself having an easy pregnancy and painless childbirth, and in doing so, involve all your senses and emotions, your mind will adopt this mindset and because of the law of attraction, you will have the pregnancy you envision. If, on the other hand, you envision a problematic pregnancy, your pregnancy will be problematic.

With that in mind, let's now discuss some easy tips that will make you have a smoother time during pregnancy.

Tips for an Easy Pregnancy

The following tips will make your pregnancy and Labor easier:

10: Perineal Massage

Most women are fearful of tearing during birth, which is when the perineum, the soft skin between the vagina and anus, tears because of the pressure placed on it as you bear down and its proximity to the vaginal canal.

While there is no guarantee that you shall not tear, various studies have concluded that regular perineal massage in the third trimester reduces chances of tearing in first time mothers over 30 years old by up to 5%.

11: Optimal Fetal Positioning

Because of inactivity and a sedentary lifestyle, gravity encourages the spine, which is the heaviest part of the baby, to roll to the back of the mother's body. This positioning (OFP) encourages the baby to get into the best position before Labor, which is facing the mother. When the baby's head presses against the mother's tailbone, the result is a slower birth coupled with immense pain.

To avoid this, spend a specific portion of time (10 minutes is enough) sitting upright with a light forward lean. Alternatively, you can kneel on the floor and lean forward into a couch. Studies suggest that if you do this every day in the last trimester (37 weeks to the onset of Labor), you will reduce the chance of your baby being in a posterior position at birth. You should start this practice early on in your pregnancy and practice it for 15 minutes twice a day.

12: Kegels

Kegels are a pelvic floor exercise that if religiously practiced all through pregnancy, will help you avoid medical interventions during childbirth. You should engage in kegels by squeezing your pelvic muscles together and holding for as a long as you can. This will make pushing your baby easier and the birth process faster.

Practical Hypnobirthing Advice for Women

Hypnobirthing has been gaining popularity worldwide for the last few years. We come across many videos and stories over the Internet, where people have shared their experiences with Hypnobirthing and how beautifully it changed their minds and helped in achieving a natural and painless birth. Hypnobirthing however needs some amount of preparation before you get into labor. The best time to begin Hypnobirthing is from 18-30 weeks. Although there are many classes available, which you can attend to learn the methods of Hypnobirthing, it may be difficult for some to attend a class or afford it. Hypnobirthing is yet to gain popularity in many countries so keeping that in mind, here are some pointers that you can follow, and practice Hypnobirthing at home. The benefits that Hypnobirthing can offer you are as follows"

- When you're breathing in the right way, you trigger your parasympathetic nervous system and that is the part of your body that make you feel calm and relaxed.

- It slows your heart rate down, which may help your baby by gently bringing your baby's heart rate down too.

- You get more oxygen for your muscles, especially the womb, which is a very powerful muscle that is helping you birth the baby.

- If you're really focused on your breathing, it is also a great distraction from what is going on around you or distraction from what is going on in your womb when you're in labor.

The sooner you start practicing the techniques of Hypnobirthing the better it is. The more you practice, the more you feel the confidence in yourself and are prepared to have a natural, calm birthing experience. Before you begin, it is essential that you read about it and gain as much knowledge as possible. Since you are doing it on your own, it will naturally take a lot of reading and listening so that you can practice it correctly. In this process it is important to involve your husband or birthing partner. They definitely play a major role in the entire process and could help you with it.

It is important to understand how Hypnobirthing works. When we are approaching labor there is something known as FTP that increases our pains. FTP stands for Fear, Tension and Pain. This increases our adrenaline and fear to such an extent that it leads to more pain. This fear can lower the blood circulation to your uterus and therefore increase your pain. That is why you need to be as calm and stress free as possible. Listening to Hypnobirthing audios and learning the correct breathing techniques can help with that. You can download audios from applications on your phone or online. If possible involve your husband while practicing Hypnobirthing.

Here are some things you need to keep in mind before starting practicing Hypnobirthing.

- Talk about your fears. Say you have a fear of tearing while giving birth or you are too worried about the extent of pain you will go through while birthing. Here you can talk to your husband about it or your mother or friend. Try and eliminate those fears from your mind and think positively.

- Listen to some relaxation audios. There are plenty of audios available online. Download them and save them on your phone and listen to them for about 20-30 minutes every single day. Since you would have been listening to your relaxation videos all throughout your last few weeks of pregnancy, it will be easier for you to relax during labor. Make sure this is practiced every single day so that you are well prepared for the big day. Best time to listen to your audios is during nap time or bedtime. Even if you fall asleep during the session, you're still listening to the audio and taking it in as our hearing senses never really rest.

- You can start with this practice from 18 weeks onwards. Many women choose to start off when they are about 25-30 weeks pregnant but what if you are above 30 weeks pregnant? There is nothing to worry. You can even begin by 35-38 weeks. It is never too late to start relaxing yourself and being ready for the most beautiful day of your life. Imagine starting your journey with your newborn in such a calm and effective manner. The essence of Hypnobirthing is that it is never too late to begin with.

- Next, it is very important that your hospital staff or your mid wife be aware that you have been practicing Hypnobirthing. You will be much calmer in labor as compared to an average woman. It may so happen that you are calm but if you are talking through your contractions, the midwives or the hospital staff may think that you are not ready and may ask you to go home. Quite often, it is not easy to breathe through or stay calm during contractions. At least that is how it has been happening for the last few decades. The midwives are accustomed to seeing women in labor howling in pain and this calmness in you may actually lead them to believe that you are still not ready when in fact you are. Therefore, it is extremely important for you or your husband to insist and to convey it to your midwife or hospital staff that you have been practicing Hypnobirthing and that you are naturally calm. It could also help to inform your midwife or doctor in advance that you are practicing Hypnobirthing. This way, they will be prepared and expect you to be calmer and more stress free as compared to any average woman in labor.

- Practicing Pregnancy Yoga or Pregnancy Pilates can be very helpful to keep your body more energized and calm during labor. Many recommend it, and a lot of women swear by it. Breathing is very important during pregnancy and especially during labor. It will help you to sleep better, and as we all know, sleeping during pregnancy can get a little uncomfortable for some and thus being able to sleep better will definitely be a boon. Practicing some Yoga moves and Pilates, can help you go through the process smoothly. It induces calmness and relaxation.

- Maintain a healthy and balanced diet. It is crucial that you have a healthy balanced diet during your pregnancy and after birth. It is fine to indulge into your cravings every once in a while, but eating junk food and something that is not great for your gut can cause a lot of discomfort. It will come in the way of your smooth sailing pregnancy hence it is important that you maintain a good balanced diet on a regular basis.

- Acupressure and relaxing massages. This is optional, but if possible and if available in your area, it is recommended that you take some acupressure and relaxing massages. If you cannot go out and get this from a professional, ask your husband to do the needful. A gentle, firm massage usually helps in relaxing you and it will release the hormone oxytocin, which is a calming hormone and will help you during labor and after labor to stimulate the milk ducts to secrete milk.

- Meditation has over the years and centuries proven to be the best method to ease you from tension and anxiety. Some people choose to focus on breathing and some choose to listen to music. There are many different ways to meditate. In this technique your body responds beautifully to visuals. You need to take time out to imagine birthing comfortably. Imagining all your muscles relaxing during pregnancy and prepare yourself mentally for your birthing experience. Through this visualization, you can create pathways in your brain that lead to subconscious responses during real life situations.

- Educating and preparing yourself before labor can leave you feeling stress free and in control. The biggest fear at this point, especially when it is your first time is the fear of the unknown. It is completely normal to feel apprehensive about the process and the journey you are about to begin. By choosing to educate and prepare yourself with something as easy and diverse as Hypnobirthing, doesn't just allow you to learn about the process of birthing and how to be in control of your body, but will also let you learn and choose different techniques to help you stay relaxed and at ease during your pregnancy, birth and after birth when the baby is born.

What Not to Do While Practicing Hypnobirthing

Do not engage into negative birth stories

In our culture, it is very common to talk about the horror stories of birthing. Most women today will tell you how horrific and traumatizing the experience was and that will eventually lead to a traumatized birthing experience for you as well. As stated above, the fear of the unknown plays the biggest role here. This is common with mothers who have had more than one pregnancy and birthing experiences as well. Since their first birthing experience was horrible and close to a nightmare, they expect the same to happen to them during their second or third birthing experience.

It is essential that you do not ponder and over think about what is going to happen. Hypnobirthing will definitely help you to overcome those fears, but you need to make a conscious effort not to indulge your mind into negative thoughts of the past or get worked up and nervous based on someone else's experience. Therefore, it is essential that you focus on all the positivity in your life and go ahead with that positive mind-frame towards your birthing.

It is not to undermine the true trauma that women have gone through, because many women have gone through severe trauma. It is unfortunately the norm today to have a birthing experience that is nothing less of a horror movie, but it is not natural. We have to surpass that thought and not allow it into our lives. What is natural is the woman is able to go innately inside to experience the powerful ability to give birth without pain.

It is difficult on a day-to-day basis to stay away from negative stories and experiences. It is unfortunately a norm to experience massive amount of pain during birthing that people somehow like to share it with other pregnant mothers, not realizing the impact it will have on their minds. If you have someone like that in your family or in your friend circle, make sure you either convey it very gently to them to not share such experiences with you or politely excuse yourself from the conversation. Negativity always attracts negativity. It is not in your hands to stop them from talking, but it is in your hands to not listen to them. Most movies or TV series also have a lot of traumatic birthing experience. You will hardly see a calm, normal water birth or hospital birth. That is not dramatic enough of the TV shows obviously, hence they always portray horrified, screaming mothers in agony. Move yourself away from the situation or just change the channel. If birthing was that bad, do you think people would have more babies?

Not looking after yourself

You need to slow down. It is natural for us to keep ourselves busy all the time. Getting the baby's crib or bedroom ready or perhaps, getting your hospital bag ready can be some of the important things you need to manage before the baby arrives, but it is important you take some time out for yourself and relax. Go swimming, take time out to pamper yourself, go on a break with your friends, take long walks and, very importantly, take lots of naps. Rest is of utmost importance here. While you are taking your naps, you can practice the various Hypnobirthing breathing exercises as well and listen to the audios.

Practical advice for the Father

Along with the mother, the father also needs to be on his toes when the baby is arriving, or has arrived. Efficiency is the key here. Prepare yourself days before the baby is born. If you are going to be with your wife or partner during her delivery, make sure that you are calm too. If you are worked up, it obviously goes against the core of Hypnobirthing. It is advisable to read up on Hypnobirthing in detail for the father as well, as that will give you more confidence and help you to stay calm and keep your partner calm too. Prepare yourself and your home before the baby arrives. Meal prep is a lifesaver. Make sure you have enough food in the house to take you through the day or week. While your partner is attending to the baby, you take responsibility of the household chores.

Instincts

Go with your instincts but trust the mother's instincts the most. A mother's instinct is very powerful. As a father, you have to believe in your partner's instincts and in yours too. A father's role is essential when it comes to Hypnobirthing. You will be the main and key point of contact between the hospital staff and your partner. You are probably thinking, she will be completely relaxed, what could go wrong? Well, truth be told, most doctors see pregnant patients who are screaming and howling in pain. For them, that is "Normal." The moment they see a patient who is calm and composed, they think that she is not ready (as she is not screaming), and probably send her back home. At this point, your role comes into to play. You have to insist that she is actually going through labor and that she is calm because she has been practicing Hypnobirthing. You have to be firm and insistent if needed. We have seen many instances where the mother is sent back home because according to the staff, she is showing no signs of labor, when in fact she is in labor.

Father's role in Hypnobirthing

It is natural to be skeptical of the whole process. You must wonder "how can I practice Hypnobirthing? Well, there are ways that you can. It is important that the father also remains calm and level headed during the birthing process. There are a number of calming audios and videos on how the father can also practice Hypnobirthing with the mother. It will help you stay focused and you can also help your partner with the breathing exercises. When she has you with her to breathe with and as a support system, it will build her confidence and perhaps make her calmer.

- Talk about your fears - Talk to your partner about your fears. Say you fear being a bad parent, or that you may not be able to stand up to your baby's expectations. Talk to your partner or talk to a friend about it. Be open about your fears, it is very natural. Having a conversation about it is very important, just like talking about your career or life choices.

- Encourage your partner to practice every day - Even if it means that you sit with your partner and encourage her and practice with her, do it. Sometimes she may not be in a mood, or just plain exhausted. You can lie down with her and practice with her. Massage her legs, shoulders or lower back to relax her and keep her calm while she practices her breathing. This will bring you closer as a couple and make your partner feel important. Your involvement will make her more confident of her life choices and pregnancy.

- At Birth – The father's main role during the birthing process is to make sure that no one disturbs the mother's private space and her aura of positivity and calm. This is important in the second stage of labor, as that is when the doctors or midwives will instruct her to push and interfere with her space.

  You can prompt her during surges. Ask her to concentrate only on your voice. She will obviously have more confidence on your instructions, as she is aware of your involvement. Your voice will help her stay focused and keep her calm. It is the father's duty to remind her to play the relaxation audios in case she has forgotten about it. During pregnancy, you can listen to the relaxation audios before you sleep as these audios not just help a pregnant woman stay calm, but also helps keep you calm. The gentle back stroking that you might have learned during pregnancy, may be of great help here and is wonderful during labor. Make sure she is not dehydrated and offer her water a few times. Giving birth is a strenuous physical and mental activity. Make sure she has some snacks available to help her keep her energy levels up. Essential oils can be used to calm the environment. A few drops on a handkerchief can promote calmness and relaxation.

- After Birth – This is the most important time out of all this. Immediately insist on skin to skin (skin contact) between the mother and the baby. They do not need to be separated, unless there is an emergency. This skin to skin will help stimulate milk production. You have to latch the baby on within a few minutes of it being born. You can also provide skin to skin to the baby as this will help in the baby-daddy bonding too.

- Continue to care – Probably the most important thing that the father can offer here is to continue to care for the mother and the child. The support you provide at this stage and stages after helps build your relationship positively. This relationship includes the bond between the Partners as well as the bond between the father and the baby. Sadly this seldom happens. The mother is left alone to do things on her own, which can lead to a lot of stress, frustration and even postpartum depression. Give her and the baby, this enormous gift of your support and help.

Breech Baby Precautions during Hypnobirthing

If you have a professional, who is an expert at Hypnobirthing, you can leave it up-to them to help you with a breech baby. However, if you have been following Hypnobirthing by yourself, you may not want to risk it and depend on your midwife to take the decision for you. It is very much possible for the midwife or the doctor to turn a breech baby into position and assist you with birthing.

In the modern world, a breech baby is automatically delivered via C-section. It has become a norm, but there are many Hypnobirthing mothers who have easily managed to deliver a breech baby without any drugs, no excess pain and in a gentle and easy manner. It is an assumption that having a baby is a medical emergency. However, a healthier and more positive assumption can be that all is well and having a positive attitude towards the entire process. We should not intervene unless it is completely necessary.

Frequently Asked Questions About Hypnobirthing

How does Hypnobirthing differ from Other Birthing procedures?

Hypnobirthing is a method where you learn to stay calm and relaxed during childbirth. Unlike other childbirth experiences where birthing is expected to be painful and scary and many women are trained and modeled to bear the pain, Hypnobirthing teaches exactly the opposite. It teaches you to stay calm and relaxed during the entire process. It teaches you that pain is a natural process during labor and that you should embrace it positively. In Hypnobirthing you understand that hormones that generate fear cause pain. They learn to release endorphins (the good hormones) instead.

The breathing technique in Hypnobirthing is what makes it different from the usual birthing technique. Shallow, abrupt and exhausting breaths can increase your anxiety and block the supply of oxygen to your body. Whereas the breathing techniques in Hypnobirthing, like the long slow and rhythmic breathing can allow you to achieve a shorter and less painful and more comfortable labor and birthing experience.

Will I remember my birthing experience? Will I be Unconscious?

Unlike the popular belief that while Hypnobirthing you will be unconscious, it is actually quite the contrary. During Hypnobirthing you are very well aware of your surroundings while being in control and contact with your body. You are the one controlling you body and managing the pain. Though you are deeply relaxed, you will often find that your experience is not distorted by anyone's presence and you are not distracted from your birthing environment and experience while you are focusing on yourself and your baby.

What if circumstances necessitate Medical intervention? Will Hypnobirthing work for me?

It is absolutely possible for Hypnobirthing to work for you if at all you are in a situation where other medical interference is mandatory. You can still make your birthing experience beautiful and filled with calmness and joy. You will find yourself more in control. Mothers who have needed C-sections due to medical reasons have recounted that they felt relaxed before, throughout and right after childbirth. They needed no extra medication and were able to return to their normal life fairly quickly.

Will I experience Pain-free Birthing experience with Hypnobirthing?

As it's said above, Hypnobirthing does not promise a pain free birthing experience, although many mothers swear that their birthing experience was as pain-free as possible and they were able to manage the pain beautifully. When the main cause of pain, i.e. fear and anxiety, is eliminated, birthing is accomplished in a much shorter span, thereby reducing labor time and increasing the comfort levels. Hypnobirthing mothers will still experience contractions and pressure, but they will learn to work with their bodies through these sensations, thus avoiding the excruciating pain everybody keeps talking about as if it's normal and expected.

How do I engage my healthcare providers in the process, if they are unaware of Hypnobirthing?

Today, more and more health care providers are becoming aware of Hypnobirthing and its benefits. Many hospitals even offer Hypnobirthing as an option in their child's birth programs. Hypnobirthing is also taught in many medical schools to student doctors. But, if your caregiver is not aware of this concept, make sure you discuss it with them much earlier in your pregnancy. Discuss the techniques you will be using and the kind of birthing environment you would prefer. Have a plan and learn how to create birth preferences, which will help you to communicate your birth goals with your health care provider, midwife or doctor. If you have taken a class, your Hypnobirthing instructor can also have a conversation with your health care provider and discuss the same in detail.

When should I start my Hypnobirthing classes during pregnancy?

Hypnobirthing is mainly a class meant to practice relaxation. You can begin a class any time but the best time would be between 18-30 weeks. Before that you can practice some breathing techniques at home just to be in the rhythm. If you start this class earlier in your pregnancy, you will have more time to practice your breathing techniques and enjoy a more relaxed and calm pregnancy as well.

Who can attend or practice a Hypnobirthing class with me?

If you choose to attend a class, your husband, partner or even mother can attend the class with you. Midwives and doula's are also usually welcome to attend it with you. It is important to have these people around, who will be your main support during pregnancy, to attend the class or practice Hypnobirthing at home with you. They will know what to expect and that it's normal to be calm and composed during labor. They will also know your breathing techniques and will be able to help you. It is not necessary for your birth companion to attend all the Hypnobirthing classes with you. It is up to you to allow them into your space and decide how much to allow them. It is not compulsory for them to practice the breathing exercises with you if they do not wish to, although it is beneficial in any life circumstances they may face in the future.

What should I bring to my Hypnobirthing class?

You will be informed about what to take with you when you attend the class but basically you need to take yourself, you companion, a book and pen to take notes and to increase your comfort you have to make sure you are dressed comfortably. You may take with you extra cushions and blankets if required. A bottle of water can be very helpful and some light snacks if required. If you are practicing Hypnobirthing by yourself at home, basically almost all of the above will be required, but obviously you will have it with you in your home at your disposal. You will just have to make sure that all your requirements are in place before beginning the session by yourself. Try not to get distracted and keep your cell phone and Television switched off. Avoid all kinds of distractions and practice.

Keep your mind frame positive and do not read or listen to any horror birthing stories. If you're attending a class, make sure you keep yourself away from such negativity and concentrate on your wellbeing and your baby's wellbeing.

Do I need to attend other prenatal classes?

It is totally up-to you to attend other classes. Hypnobirthing class will provide you with information on breathing techniques and how to have a natural and pain-free birth. Other classes will teach you the other important things; mainly what comes after the baby is born. It will cover information on complications and unwanted interventions. Gaining more information on birthing and after care will only help you to take an informed decision. They cover topics such as cord clamping, role of the partner in baby caring, breastfeeding etc.

What if I have had a C – section in my first pregnancy and want to attempt natural birthing in the second? Is it possible? Will Hypnobirthing help?

Absolutely. Hypnobirthing will definitely help you to take an informed and more confident decision. Many women have been able to deliver normally, even after having a c–section the first time around. It will help you stay calm and focused.

Hypnobirthing, as you know, is meant to make you feel calm and relaxed. Many people mistake Hypnobirthing for water birthing or some sort of hippie birthing experience. At the end of a Hypnobirthing class or a session at home, you will feel much more confident, relaxed and more in control of your body. You do not have to be dependent on your Doctors or midwives to make decisions for you. With Hypnobirthing, you realize that you do not have to experience a painful and traumatic birth. You can be much more relaxed and release all the anxieties you may have about birthing or even your past birthing experiences. It lets you discover the joy and beauty of a birth rather than the dreaded trauma you would usually be prepared for or experience if you hadn't practiced Hypnobirthing.

Hypnobirthing doesn't mean that you'll be in a trance or hypnotized while practicing. It simply means that you will be in a state of relaxation and composure, almost as if hypnotized but the only difference is, you are in control of your body, surroundings and decisions.

Hypnobirthing has no religious or cultural boundaries to it. It is simply a way of birthing that is now becoming more and more popular throughout the world. Some Mothers are very skeptical of this practice, mainly if they have already experienced a horrific first delivery, until they experience Hypnobirthing for themselves.

In short, Hypnobirthing makes your birthing experience calm and relaxed. It rids you of all your inhibitions and anxiety and makes you more confident and in control of your body exactly how nature intended it to happen.

Challenges in Pregnancy & How to overcome those challenges

Pregnancy is a beautiful journey. The experience of your body changing, the feel of your tummy growing, the kicks and movements in your womb are some of the most ecstatic feelings in the world, but it not always a bed of roses for many. The challenges we encounter during pregnancy are many and can get extremely difficult to handle, but there are ways you can do it.

Morning sickness

Morning sickness is one of the most common challenges that you may face during pregnancy. It usually goes away by the end of the first trimester but, for some, it may continue until the end of the third trimester. Morning sickness can happen any time during the day (although it is termed as morning sickness) and so, if you are facing this problem, you can find ways to make it more tolerable. Some of the ways that you can ease out your morning sickness are:

- Eat little, but often throughout the day. An empty stomach may create acidity in your stomach and thus make you more uncomfortable.

- Avoid foods that can trigger your morning sickness

- Drink water in between your meals

- Get plenty of rest

- Lemon is usually proven to help with morning sickness.

- Cold meals are more helpful than hot meals

- Ginger tea is a good antioxidant and helps to keep morning sickness at bay.

- Try alternate therapy like a massage.

- Exercise while you can. Keeping yourself active will help distract your mind and help with morning sickness.

- Talk to a friend who has gone through the same. Having someone face the same challenges, as you can be very comforting.

Heartburn/Reflux –

Heartburn or reflux is also a very common problem during pregnancy. Unfortunately it gets worse at the end of the pregnancy. It is described as a burning sensation in the throat and stomach and usually accompanied by chest tightness, nausea and acidity in the mouth. Herbal teas may help to bring down the heartburn. Talk to your doctor and ask him to prescribe an anti acidity medicine.

Problems sleeping:

This is the most common problem pregnant women face. As your belly grows bigger, very few sleeping positions get you comfortable and a good night's sleep. The best solution in such a situation is pillows. Use as many pillows as possible to sleep. Using pillows just under your back or to rest your belly on can be immensely helpful to get some well deserved good night's sleep. Now days there are different kinds of pregnancy pillows also available that can be used to sleep comfortably but, in all honesty, simple regular pillows also work equally well.

Foot and back massages work wonders. Just the fact that you are relaxed and all the right pressure points on your body are released, is enough for you to release some amount of endorphins, which is a hormone that can help relive you from stress and anxiety.

Practicing Hypnobirthing can also be a great way to ensure a good night's sleep. Some of the rituals that need to be followed while you practice Hypnobirthing involve listening to relaxing, calming music while you are getting ready for bed. It reduces your stress and anxiety levels that in turn ensures and induces peaceful and undisturbed sleep.

Cramps:

Cramps are common during pregnancy, especially in the legs, due to all the extra weight you are carrying. You body is also losing nutrients due to the growing baby because of which you need to ensure a good healthy meal along with your multivitamins.

Eating food that is high in magnesium and calcium can help with the cramps. Drink a lot of water to keep your muscles hydrated.

When you know you are cramping, flex your foot and massage the area that is cramping.

Make sure you are always wearing comfortable shoes. Exercise also helps to reduce cramping episodes.

Hypnobirthing can help with this as well, as the breathing exercises ensure circulation of oxygen throughout your body, which will definitely help with blood flow circulation that in turn will reduce the cramps.

Back Pain:

Back pain is also a very common discomfort many women face while they are pregnant. The back take a lot of pressure from the growing belly and the shape of your backbone also changes. Due to the change in this anatomy, pain is usually inevitable.

If your pain is chronic, it is best advised to talk to your doctor. However, if your pain is bearable, you can ask your partner to massage your back and relieve you from the pain. Simple oil massages help tremendously. Again, exercises can also help here. By providing your body with the needed circulation and stretch, back pains can easily be managed.

Although all these problems arise during pregnancy and many are inevitable, it is still a very beautiful experience. We have so many techniques and tricks to overcome them today, which in turn make these problems very small as compared to the birth of the tiny human inside your body. It is extremely important to have a positive attitude throughout your pregnancy. Stay away from negativity and horror stories (as stated in Hypnobirthing) and create an environment of peace and tranquility around you. It is understandable that there are some situations that are not in our hands and we can get stressed with the surroundings, but for the sake of our baby, we need to look at the bigger picture and control the outcome.

Conclusion

We have come to the end of the book. Thank you for reading and congratulations for reading until the end.

Hypnobirthing, while a relatively new concept in modern day society, is something women since time immemorial, have been using to have easy and happy pregnancies and pain free births.

As you embark on the journey to bringing your child into this world in the way nature intended—naturally—educate yourself, break free from the fear of pregnancy pain, and practice the tips from section 3 to have a happy and positive pregnancy.

If you found the book valuable, can you recommend it to others? One way to do that is to post a review.

Thank you and good luck!

Dr. Melissa Keane